AUTISM &
ASPERGER

All You Need to Know About Asperger
Syndrome & Autism.

BY

KENNETH D. MOORE

TABLE OF CONTENT

CHAPTER 1

INTRODUCTION

It so important that we learn as much as we can about this Asperger Syndrome, and when dealing with previously diagnosed cases (either self or others) know what should be done to manage, control and help live through it well.

Asperger Syndrome is with a collection of mental disorder that attack persons of diverse races all over the world. It's grouped as part of Autism Spectrum Disorder (ASD).

This "Asperger Syndrome" can be either chronic and last for as long as one lives or just for very many years, and affects both sexes of humans; although researches have revealed that males are by some proportion likely to suffer this mental disorder than females.

In this book you shall find exhaustive explanation of things you may want to know better concerning Asperger management practices and new ideas of range of tested treatments method and directions on resolving which will work and how to decide on what treatment method to follow.

Follow this book with patience and open mindedness and discover amazing information on management measures and precautionary steps.

Parents, nurses, guardians, teachers etc. you never can tell when someone close may need your help.

Save a Life, Even Yours!

CHAPTER 2

DETAILS ON ASPERGER

Asperger Syndrome is a group of Autism Spectrum Disorder (ASD) that deters mental orderliness of a person or persons. This in turn distress the communication and socializing skill of the individual(s).

Previously, Asperger Syndrome was cared for as a disease or disorder of its own, until further research showed that it can well be diagnosed as part of Autism. Hence people, mainly children who show these signs are diagnosed and treated as autistic.

Autism as a disorder describes a case of 'mental developmental disorder that fluctuate in overall characteristics. A number of these states of developmental disorder, typically banking on the weightiness include Autistic Tendencies, Pervasive Developmental Disorder, High functioning or low functioning, etc. are terms used to elucidate the behaviors of children (mostly), that falls into the Autism Spectrum.

Most children diagnosed with Asperger Syndrome are famous to be among the High-Functioning Autism Spectrum, and likely to affect boys than girls.

Among them are children who are intelligent in purpose but find it difficult to speak or write properly. This people have comparable symptoms as Asperger, and are called Social Pragmatic Interaction Disorder.

CHAPTER 3

CHARACTERISTICS ASSOCIATED WITH ASPERGER SYNDROME

Below are some known characteristics noticed among children with Asperger Syndrome:

- Complexity socializing
- Complexity communicating
- Obsessions about picky topics or things
- Small facial looks
- Odd speech patterns
- Odd signs
- Complexity understanding body languages

- Engaging in unnecessary headstrong routines
- Exhibition of weird sensitivity to stimuli. For instance e.g. having issues with sounds that others can hardly hear or cover ears to keep out sounds from the surrounding.
- Children who are suffering from Asperger Syndrome can function on average as everyone else in their daily routine, the exceptions being that they show signs of social immaturity
- They communicate well with people older than with their age mates.
- Motor delays in their actions.
- Abnormal nervousness
- Awkwardness
- No or low interest in things.
- Difficulty showing empathy for others (mostly among adults with Asperger Syndrome)

As said earlier, Asperger Syndrome all through one's lifetime and with new characters relating at some points. Good and quick intervention can go a long way in relieving the excesses that might be related with this disorder.

CHAPTER 4

SIGNS AND SYMPTOMS

It is imperative that children/ individuals be taken to a specialist for appraisal and appropriate diagnosis of Asperger Syndrome or Attention Deficit Hyperactivity Disorder (ADHD). Even more is the need for a parent or guardian to be able to detect that something is unusual.

Below are some signs and symptoms a child suffering from Asperger Syndrome could show:

a. Creepy behaviors or mannerisms.

b. presence of no common sense.

c. Odd movements.

d. Unsocial behaviors

e. Self centeredness and never talking of benefits of others.

f. Meager cognitive verbal and nonverbal skills.

g. Abnormal repetition of speech.

h. Poor reading and writing skills.

i. Obsession with complicated subjects.

Note: most children with Asperger Syndrome usually do not have issues with language development like those with autism. Even with their good vocabulary development skills, many among them habitually have language disorder. They also are intelligent and have normal coherent development but may show trouble organizing and focusing.

CHAPTER 5

POSSIBLE CAUSES

There has been no exact cause or reason associated to Asperger Syndrome and Autism as Mental Health Professionals and Researchers are still working on it.

Below are some facts about Asperger Syndrome:

- The abnormalities of the brain can be one sure cause of Asperger Syndrome, as disparity in functions and structures have been dicovered during sophisticated brain photography.

- Asperger Syndrome may be transferred through the gene as it might be linked with other Mental Health issues.
- Asperger Syndrome cannot be caused by any manner of emotional denial or upbringing, as they are sometimes confused.

CHAPTER 6

DIAGNOSIS

There's a possibility of parents mistaking Asperger Syndrome for normal behavioral disparity, as they may function well in some areas of life; consequently making diagnosis difficult.

Only a specialized personnel in this field can diagnose any form of abnormality, by doing a critical asking about symptom's history, motor skills development, language pattern, activities, distractions, abnormal habits, etc.

More attentions are given to social development (issues with social communications and relationships).

Make sure to see a doctor for assistance, who in turn will refer you to a specialist when you notice any of the symptoms similar to those above.

a. **Psychiatrist:** specialized in the care and treatments of Mental Health conditions.

b. **Psychologist:** specializes in diagnosing, caring and treating emotion and behavior related issues.

c. **Development Pediatrician:** specializes in speech, language and other developmental crisis.

d. **Pediatric Neurologist:** specializes in all brain related situations.

It's pertinent to know that more than one doctor may have to see the child for more accurate results and know that the following questions may come up:

a. Is the kid welcoming, and how well does the child relate with people?

b. Does he show abnormal center of attention on a particular activity or subject?

c. What symptoms did you notice the child have and when they started?

d. When did your child first speak and how?

CHAPTER 7

TREATMENTS & MAAGEMENTS

For now, there are no known treatments for Asperger Syndrome. Children will have to grow into adulthood with the Syndrome and eventually maximize their lives when they have support and good education.

Behaviors and characteristics can differ from one child to another with Asperger Syndrome. It's now for the specialist to resolve how best to go about the therapy and what style to apply.

Treatments may include:

1. **Cognitive behavioral therapy (CBT):** this will support and aid the child's pattern of thinking and gain some level of emotional control. He may be able to control repetitions, outbursts, obsessions and meltdowns at the end of the therapy.

2. **Applied behavior analysis:** this supports and aid o develop better social and relating skills in the child. The therapist will have to decide whether to praises or take on other "positive reinforcement" to get results.

3. **Parental training and education:** it's important that parents be trained on methods to be competently relate and teach one with Asperger Syndrome.

4. **Speech-language therapy:** This will support and develop the communication skills of the child. He will be taught to speak normally, gesticulate and make eye contacts.

5. **Social skills training:** The therapist may introduce the child to a group and

demonstrate to him/her how to better communicate with others. It's easier to learn this way most times.

6. **Medications:** at this time, there are no known or approved medications to cure Asperger or autism; but they only minimize symptoms like anxiety.

Some medical doctors may recommend these:

a. Antipsychotic medicines.

b. Stimulants

c. Selective serotonin reuptake inhibitors (SSRIs).

It's vital to connect as much caregivers as possible. That is, that everyone (teachers, doctors, etc.) should be very involved with the child's development.

All these worked with and the child will be able to lead a good life like any other person.

CHAPTER 8

NECESSARY SUPPORTS FOR ASPERGER SYNDROME PATIENTS

Here are some of the sure ways you can be of aid and backing to a child with Asperger Syndrome:

a. Assist the child become self confident and autonomous; these will help the child's life later.

b. Treat the child with enough respect as you give others; nothing less.

c. Ask the help of other caregivers, not just for the kid but for yourself (parent, teacher) as well. You must be well to be able to take care of another. Go for regular checkups.

d. Prepare and train yourself particularly to be ready for the tasks ahead.

e. Learn to be everything to the child; teacher, doctor, and friend. And always act with the child's development at heart.

f. Find a management or intercession program that suits your child. Autism Society of America (ASA) advices that you speak with those in charge of programs to be sure they can meet the child's special needs.

CHAPTER 9

FINALLY BE ENCOURAGED

Children who live with Asperger Syndrome go either the usual schools or special schools. While the later may be costlier, but the formal needs lots of supports and back-ups from teachers, parents etc. to encourage them on.

There are known cases of people living with Asperger Syndrome who have lived remarkably well in the past; and so can your child.

It's therefore wise to advice you do not give up on your child because he/she was diagnosed with Asperger Syndrome. Help is closer than you think.

THE END